How to Lose Weight After 40!

50 Ways to Lose Weight Now!

By: Rosemary Hershey

"How Can You Lose Weight After 40?" Well, let me count the ways because there are at least 50 from which you can choose every day that will bring you closer to losing than gaining.

Imbedded in these nifty fifty, is a winning strategy that will rub off almost unnoticed in the mix of your everyday life and give you what you don't have now, a winning platform to lose your weight permanently!

A platform of change because the diet story most women follow fails to keep the weight off leading right back to where it all started, overeating and weight gain. It sucks and you need to change the dynamics of a failed process into a lifestyle that works for you.

Diets are all about your weight, how you eat, what you eat, when and where you eat but blank on why you eat. You already know how to diet, you already know how to lose weight, but what you don't know is why you can't keep it off.

The key to your freedom is self-knowledge and discovering how to create solutions that end your war with self, with food and with your body. You can have it all without losing it all when you know why you're in trouble.

Trouble? War? What war?

Do I really mean war? You may cringe at the idea but, yes, it's about war! Yours.

The issue is the life you have and the life you want, it's about the body you have and the body you want, it's about your victories and about your defeats, all relationship based, it's how you live and don't live, it's who you are and wish you could be, fought through the haven or the hell of food. Time to change those definitions, agreed?

It's easier than you think. In fact, all you have to do to change your life is make the decision.   Once you choose to stop repeating diets and take control of your own life, it happens. Once you start trusting in yourself by keeping your word, by promising only what you can deliver, and then doing it, you build your faith. Over time, your credibility deepens, you never give up even when it's one step forward and two steps back, you stay the course refusing to abandon the life you want, and your world improves.

Your transformation starts here, with step 1.

Do step 1 faithfully and even if you do nothing else, that one action alone will change your life.

"Unless you change the things you do, nothing changes."

--Albert Einstein

Rosemary Hershey.

<u>50</u> Ways to Lose Weight Now!

One. <u>Create a contract with yourself.</u>

Contract? Yes, a written contract with yourself that treats your word as if it means something, a contract that holds you accountable to achieve your intentions and expects that you will do all that you have promised to do.

Date it, from you to you, and put yourself out there on paper to memorialize your new commitment and the power of your words:

"*I, Mary Louise Adams, promise to hold myself accountable to keep my word in all matters, big and small.*

This is my contract with myself because I understand and agree that my word matters. I am committed to honor it because my word is my bond and my integrity. I <u>will</u> live my best effort in keeping my promises."

Your contract is your law and it implies your commitment to perform with integrity and do your best, regardless of outcomes.

Write your contract and put your mind on notice that you mean business and will not quit on yourself.

What can you promise yourself to help change your life?

What can you commit to and deliver on?

2. **Make your promises simple**. Don't overreach.

3. **Make it realistic. Always ask yourself, "Is it doable?" Be honest with yourself and your expectations. Ask again, "Will I do this, at this time?" If in doubt, leave it out.**

4. **Write it down.**

5. **Answer these no-fluff questions**. Add your own.

   a. "Why do I want to lose weight?" List 6 reasons.

   b. "What do I expect or want from this change?" How will it make me feel?

(a)Examples: self growth, stronger relationships, self power, self validation, more respect inside and outside, healthier.

(b)Examples: noticed, respected, confident, attractive.

c. "Why do I want that feeling?" (improved self-worth? Etc)

d. "What will it bring to my life that is missing now? (power, security, balance)

e. "Why don't I have this now?" (complacency, laziness, fear)

f. What are the obstacles to my success? (overwhelm, meaningless diversions like t.v., phone chatter, internet)

g. What has stopped you or derailed you in the past? Stress, mindless eating, boredom, exhaustion, overwhelm, worry, drinking, fear, lack.

h. What lessons can you observe from your obstacles and how will you use that information to succeed now?

(g) <u>Example:</u>

Boredom: if you are bored, what can you do about it? What are some activities you could take on to invigorate your life? How can you stimulate and motivate yourself to right action? What do you enjoy? Love? Are you living it? If not, why not? Jot down some thoughts, ideas. It's a beginning. Do it.

(g) <u>Example:</u>

Tired: Learn to recognize your body signals. When you are tired, get some rest rather than a snack. Do the right thing for yourself and instead of responding with food, pause and reflect on how you are feeling. Acknowledge being tired.

What's going on in your body? How is it feeling? What does it need?

Your body is trying to tell you something so take the time to ask it and listen to it. Don't confuse your signals; don't eat to stay awake.

6. **Give yourself focused attention and reflection**. Do it.

   What's working for you?

   What's not working for you?

   Why don't you change it? Rearrange it? Do it differently?

   Take one action. Make one improvement and go from there

   with baby steps that keep get you into action, right action.

7. **Write out three small, manageable, achievable goals.**

   Think from the perspective of cause; What habits cause

   you the most grief? What goals can you write that will

   shift your habit to any degree that is positive? Start.

   Work on habit reform goals vs. weight goals. There's no

   point in simply losing weight without changing the habit

   attached to the weight. Keep it simple.

8. Frame each goal around these questions:

"What habit would I like to change most?"

"What is it I am trying to accomplish?"

(example: end noshing every night or replace high

impact treats with healthier choices.

Less t.v. and mindless eating, etc.)

"What's necessary to accomplish it?"

(Pay attention to myself, raise my awareness, learn

discernment by asking myself questions that matter.)

What's the motive behind asking questions? To uncover more of

yourself. To get to know and understand yourself and what

drives your behavior. You can't help yourself if you don't know

yourself. That's it. Questions to unravel some of your

packaging so you can get to know yourself instead of avoiding or

ignoring yourself and what is driving your life.

"I can teach anybody to get anything they want.

The problem is I can't find anybody who can tell me

what they want."   --Mark Twain

Allow yourself time to change. You need time to adapt because change is a process that takes repetition, stamina and patience. It's par for everyone and how people operate.

9. **Think about your life.**

   Describe yourself on your best days and how you feel.

   What makes life different for you on your best days and why?

   How do you get to best?

   What has to happen for you to feel your best?

   Why are you able to eat smartly when you are "on" a diet but not after the diet ends? What is the magic diet ingredient or mindset that fortifies you to behave and why can't you apply that same magic to your behavior in the "off" diet mode?

10. **What do you want? Right now? Why don't you have it?**

   Describe actions you can take to help you eat smarter, make smarter choices, make better decisions, not just occasionally, but all the time.

   If you don't want to be unhappy, decide what makes you happy.

How can you create what makes you happy?

How can you create what makes you feel good?

Get to know yourself so you can help yourself. You don't know what you don't know!

Clearly define what you are about so you can focus on working in your own best interest.   You have to know yourself to help yourself.

> *"Knowing is not enough; we must apply;*
>
> *willing is not enough, we must do."*
>
> **--Johann Wolfgang von Goethe**

11. **When are you most vulnerable?**

    (Hint --watching television, stress, overwhelm, social events, free food samples, all you can eat places, tired, holidays, alone.) Make a list of your weak links in order to prepare.

12. **Upgrade your awareness**.

    If you mindlessly eat, what will get you to notice it? What can you do to upgrade self-awareness? Write down ideas and experiment, look for solutions. For instance:

Try being your own mirror. Look at yourself as an observer and not as a critic. Review your behavior each night, and if you are unhappy with yourself, decide what you can do about changing it. What one specific behavior do you want to alter this month? Pick one you can handle now and decide how you will start. Write it down.

What can you do differently?

Think how you can alter, shift, outsmart, avoid, or redesign any behavior that does not serve you. Start on any issue but start. Realize there is always some action you can take, no matter how small or seemingly insignificant. If it moves you forward, towards the behavior you want, it's a step in the right direction. Remember that.

Learn from what does not work for you. Ask yourself what you learned about a particular situation even if you lost control to overeating. Extract the lesson, what did you get or learn from the event that will strengthen your future. If something or someone makes you feel powerless, acknowledge it and either avoid it until you are stronger, or change it. Trade entrapment for empowerment!

Example: if you can't resist stuffing yourself at all you can eat venues, avoid them until you have enough management power to handle it.

Example: If you eat through half a large bag of chips watching television before realizing it, don't buy those giant size bags. Buy individual size servings that limit portion size. Sure you can eat a 2nd or 3rd bag, but that requires awareness and changes the dynamics from mindless to intentional.

a. **Program yourself to ask questions** which lead to self-discovery and self-awareness.

Questions to ask:

"Does this action bring me closer to my goal or further away?"

"Will eating this change anything?"

"What do I want?"

Ask your own questions and sharpen your awareness.

b. **Keep a journal of your results**. If your actions flopped, why?   What can you do differently to get a better result?

c. **What did you learn** from what didn't work? What was your lesson and how can you use it to improve results next time? If you succeeded in overcoming a temptation or minimizing it, what was done differently?

If you feel trapped by a toxic situation, person, event or attachment, ask yourself what action will change or alter the dynamics, no matter how slightly, so you can better manage your life without running to food for relief. There's always something you can do so go ahead, take action. Plan.

Action puts you in power. It's empowering, proactive and necessary to create the changes you want because unless you change the things you do, nothing changes.

> *"We are what we repeatedly do. Excellence then is not an act, but a habit."*   *--Aristotle*

13. **Below are some action tips** to make change happen right now to help you lose weight.

- Start walking.

- Take the stairs.

- Join the YMCA and use their pool and/or gym.

- Join a health club and workout.

- Start a walking club with friends, neighbors, co-workers.

- Take 15-minute breaks twice a day and do a walk about.

- Get up during commercials and stretch and walk around.

- Get up at the office and walk around.

- Start a dog-walking club.

- Dance at home to your favorite music

- Learn tap dancing or fake it but get your legs moving.

- Jog

- Play tennis

- Play golf

- Jump rope.

- Park away from your destination and walk.

- Get off the bus or train one stop early and walk.

- Park away from your grocery store and walk.

- Carry your grocery bags to your vehicle or to your home.

- Hire a personal trainer online or join a group.

- Mow the lawn.

- Sweep the yard.

- Paint a room in your residence.

- Go hiking.

- Ride a bike.

- Go backpacking.

- Learn martial arts.

- Yoga

- Karate

- Do aerobics

- Lift weights

- Move. Take action. Start small but start.

- Go rock-climbing

- Learn boxing

- Get moving. If you don't use it, you lose it and that goes for flexibility, agility, vigor, vitality and overall feelings of achievement. Fight sedentary by staying active even if you don't feel like it. Activity brings rewards that include

- better sleep, better can do attitude, more self-pride and self-respect.

Practice habit-buster solutions to 8 common behaviors:

14. **Habit: Shop when hungry and food impulse buy**.

    Solution:

    Eat beforehand just enough to take the edge off.

    Fresh fruit.

    One KFC corn on the cob no butter,

    One tablespoon of peanut butter with 2 small crackers.

    Quarter pound of roast beef rolled up like a stick no bread.

    Quarter pound of turkey breast rolled up, plain, no bread.

    KFC grilled chicken leg, skinned.

    Pouch packed water based tuna 4 oz.

    Cup of no-fat cottage cheese.

15. **Habit: Skip meals and overeat later**.

    Solution: Don't skip meals.

    Realize losing weight is not about starving yourself, it's about

    building balance in your life so you can have it all without

    losing it all.

Work on portion control and foods that fill you up without being calorie dense. Desserts are not your friend here.

Skip butter, eat bread at one meal only, no fried foods, no sodas eat smaller portions, or half portions, no seconds, leaner meats, skinned chicken, steamed sides, dressings, gravies on the side.

Identify hunger vs. cravings. Ask yourself:

"Am I hungry?" Listen to your body for the answer.

Not hungry? Then decide to do without it. Take control.

16. **Habit: Buy junk food for my family I can't resist eating.**

   Solution:

Shop with a list and upgrade your food choices from junk and gunk to go but slow. You can allow treats that are fun to eat but choose healthier foods that include baked over fried. Go but slow means you can say yes to yourself with conditions. The condition is caution, a bright yellow light, proceed and be agreeable to stop. Be agreeable to set up a limit beforehand and keep your word and stop when your limit has been eaten.

Eat low fat or no fat baked chips, ditto low to no fat crackers, natural plain nuts like almonds, filberts, walnuts, pecans and buy in pre-measured small packages not giant bags. Yes to no fat pretzels, natural baked vegetable chips, low or no fat Triscuits, Wheat Thins, Matzos or Melba toast, to name a few.

Read product labels and know your stuff. Educate yourself. Limit portion size with 1oz. bags that are sold in every supermarket and are also featured at places like Starbucks.

Yes, you pay more but you're worth it because you won't mindlessly eat your way through oversized bags of treats and then beat yourself up with guilt. Stay in control.

Individual bags create accountability. You remain aware of portion size when you finish one bag and contemplate opening another, no surprises there. You can't hide under the banner of mindless eating. It's a focused choice that you make knowing there are consequences.

17. **Habit: Visit all you can eat restaurants and lose control.**

Solution:

Avoid no restraint restaurants and social events, if possible because it is an invitation to gluttony, pure and simple. An excuse to overindulge and mindlessly eat simply because you can and with everyone else doing it too, it's comfortable.

It encourages greedy behavior and the hidden side of greed is that it hides strong fears of lack; there's never enough. Greed camouflages beliefs rooted in distrust in the law of abundance. It's seeing the world from a place of lack. Lack is a negative root.

Resist all you can eat venues. And if that's not possible for some reason, then eat something substantial beforehand so you are not hungry and make a promise to yourself that you will not double dip and keep your word.

18. **Habit: Love free food samples in the supermarket.**

Solution:

Rethink free. Nothing is free. Think about it. If it takes 3500 calories to gain or lose each pound, aren't these nibbles included in the count?

There's nothing free about it. It costs you plenty not only in the calories you have no way of assessing but in the direction it leads you. Everything either moves you towards your goal and dreams or takes you further away.

If your goal is to get healthy and lose weight, how does noshing an unknown amount of calories get you there? It doesn't.

You either move in the right direction or wrong direction and nothing in between. Everything counts and everything matters in moving you forward or away so don't choose unwisely for a micro minute of pleasure.

The big picture of your life flows from those small choices made at the grocery store, or in the mall, or dining out, or eating home, or socializing, or cleaning house, or doing chores or at fast food places. Every choice creates your life and impacts the whole of your life. So the mindless snack adds its footprint to your life canvas. It matters.

19. Habit: Don't read food labels. They are too confusing.

Solution:

Buy a book on nutrition and read it. Go on the internet for help. Ask Google or Yahoo Answers and remember to keep it simple. The government offers free information via the Department of Health and there's free tips from Prevention.com as well. Ask your doctor, call your hospital For reference material from their dietician, ask your librarian, but ask and educate yourself. It's your responsibility.

Here's my brief outline for keeping it simple. It's not exact, it's not scientific, it may not even be accurate but it's a guideline that works for me when I'm mentally assessing my choices and it's impact in my life.

My Guideline:

20.   **Check servings size**. If its 3.5 servings per can or bottle, round it down to 3. Make it easy. Check calories. Let's say 100 calories per serving with 3 servings per can, all of it is 300 calories.

21.   **Check fat content**. The can says 9 grams per serving so the entire product is 27 grams of fat. (3servings x 9grams per serving.) Every fat gram contains 9 calories. The 27 total fat grams in the can multiplied by 9 means a total of 243 calories in the product is fat and out of 300 in the entire can, it's a lot. Almost 80% fat.

22.   **Check sugar content**. The product has 19 grams of sugar per serving and there are 3 servings. So 19 x 3 equals 57grams total. Every 4 grams is one teaspoon of sugar. So 57 grams divided by 4 means there are 19 teaspoons of sugar potentially in your body from one food item. It's shocking to realize through reading food labels how much sugar is in our food.

23. **Sodium content** is in milligrams per serving and the recommended daily maximum is 2000mg. When you read food labels, it's easy to conclude that we are salting our bodies to hazardous levels. Some foods and soups are so heavily salted they would account for more than half your daily dose in only one serving. Some restaurant servings are over 3500 milligrams of sodium in one meal.

How do I know? I ask for the nutritional values which many restaurants now post and make my choices from that information.

Be mindful of sodium as it affects how you feel and look.

Blood pressure spikes and our bodies experience weight gain, bloating, swollen eyes, thickened waist, and tight rings. If you experience morning after sluggishness, think salt overload!

24.   Habit: Eat fast food or restaurant meals several times a week and it's hard to eat healthy.

Solution:

Try compromise when ordering fast food meals.

If you order fried foods, remove the fried batter, blot the fries.

Some options, other than fried foods:

Try <u>baked</u> chicken at Kentucky Foods or Burger King's grilled Chicken sandwich, order dry, dressing on the side.

For those times when you can't resist the fries, compromise. Eat half. Toss the rest.

Ditto the bun with your sandwich or burger, throw out the top and enjoy your open face meal with half the carbohydrates and fewer calories.   You know what, you will hardly miss it.

Order restaurant dishes that come with gobs of sauces, dressings, seasonings, gravy, butter or barbeque all on the side.   Request your food plain and drizzle the topping on yourself for a lot less fat, calories and carbohydrates.

You will find a little goes a long way because all these dishes with sauces are big on flavor so you don't need much. Don't sit there on the receiving end of some restaurant's indiscriminate pour. You take control and dab it on your food. This includes special sauces for your burger or sandwich. Get sauces, etc. on the side. Toast dry with butter on the side. Resist desserts. Order angel food cake with fresh fruit on top.

25. **Habit: I nibble when I'm on the phone or watching t.v. or at my desk at work. I don't pay attention and before I know it, I've downed hundreds of calories.**

Solution:

Make an agreement with yourself in writing. A contract starting today to run for 30 days. The contract states that you measure what you eat by either buying individual size portions or by counting or dividing the snack into 1oz. serving size.

Keep your word and do this for 30 days and you have laid the ground work for a new habit that gives you total awareness of your actions and eliminates mindless eating. Get guidance from the label, 8 chips = 1 oz. or 8 servings per package divided into 8 slices or portions. Use common sense but measure.

Why does it matter how you think about diet?

Every day you support your body by feeding it and what and how you feed it reflects whether you are in harmony with your life or not. Your day-to-day lifestyle is your diet and your choices matter.

You didn't wake up suddenly one day overweight, did you? Of course not, so how did it happen? Think about it? It happened a little at a time, over time, from one decision at a time.

Bottom line, you are always fully responsible for the fueling your body, keeping it healthy and in shape. It's not what you do now and then after you've run amuck, it's what you do every day that brings on amuck.

Use the power of one rule.

26.   How do you eat an elephant? One piece at a time.

Think one-piece rule about losing weight. Think one small goal, one improvement each day, one choice for the right outcome, one idea about how to have a good day.

27.   Don't think diet, think food management.

Work on one weight management issue at a time. If it's a large issue or deeply engrained habit, don't tackle the whole thing at one time, learn to divide and conquer. Divide big issues into small parts then go after and conquer one part at a time. Make one improvement and feel great about it; one today, added to another tomorrow and another next week, pretty soon it's significant shifts in behavior and all of it is taking you in the right direction.

It's the eat an elephant one-piece rule.

28.   Exercise micro thinking, right now thinking.

What you eat now, in the moment, matters. Not just the plan for cutting back later or tomorrow or after the weekend, but your now choice. Cut back now.

29.   Be reasonable with your expectations and self-demands.

Try for soft-core triumphs every day; cut down or improve one thing every day.

30.   Be aware of your self-talk. Your attitude matters.

You need to treat yourself as you would treat a friend, a family member, your spouse or significant other, someone you dearly love, respect, and would never want to hurt. Why can't that friend be you? Don't judge. Don't criticize. Don't be harsh or unkind or intolerant. Observe yourself only for the purpose of learning about yourself. Accept what's done is done and agree to work on self-improvement and move on. Keep adding small improvements and remember it. Write it down each day. Read it each day, often. Today I resisted xx, I gave up soda, I won another round and resisted the cake. Etc. etc.

Write yourself a love letter and carry it with you, tape it to your refrigerator and over the places where you store food. Read it when in temptation, turmoil or distress or any time, just read it.

"Every time you smile at someone, it is an action of love, a gift to that person, a beautiful thing." –Mother Teresa

Give love to yourself in a smile and in words.

Tell yourself today and every day:

*"**Today** I will treat myself with dignity and respect.*
No name calling, no self directed anger or judgments. "

*"**Today** I will do my best and I'm good with my best, whatever that is."*

*"**Today** I will honor myself and be my best friend. I deserve loving self-support."*

*"**Today** I reject trash talk from anyone or for anyone. I do not give or accept judgments, critiques, gripes or complaints about what's wrong, what's lacking, what's hard, what's different. I love it or leave it.*

<u>LOVE LETTER TO YOURSELF</u>

Dear Mary Smith,

Although we don't communicate much lately, I want you to know how I feel because you are the most important person in the world to me.

First, I'm sorry that you have chosen not to create a more empowering life for yourself by falling silent when I call out for help. You look elsewhere to end your issues when you and I could take anything on together.

I'm upset that you are unwilling to keep yourself in better shape. It makes me sad to feel your frustration, knowing you are not giving your best or doing your best to love and respect your body, mind and spirit.

I'm so disappointed that you find excuses for your laziness and defer blame on everything outside you when the problem stems from inside you. If you spend time with me, you could identify your ache and we could action the right kind of help together.

It's troubling to watch your mood fluctuate up and down, depending on your weight and then find you chasing more false start diets which don't speak to me and don't change you.

I'm afraid of the bad things potentially affecting your health because you throw caution to the wind when eating. How could you ignore the warning signals of unhealthy eating from too much fat, too much sodium, too much sugar and too much food! Do you want to destroy me?

I'm distressed that you feel so hurt, or so lost, or so unimportant that you won't organize and discipline your life to take actions that serve you and me.

Why don't you care when I love you so much?

I want you to care. I want you to feel good about yourself. I want you to love the beautiful gift you have, your life. I want you to live your best, fully in synch with your heart's desires.

Don't fold to your fears of change when there's nothing real to fear. Come to me, I want you to be happy. I am here for you, ready and willing to be your friend. I long to help you, if you will only ask me, visit me and talk to me.

I love you and believe in you. I care so deeply for you and want you to care about me too. Can I count on that caring?

Your Loving Heart,

Mary Smith

31.   Educate yourself. Learn. Grow.

"*Pity the man who has a favorite restaurant but not a* favorite author. He's picked out a favorite place to feed his body but he doesn't have a favorite place to feed his mind."
--Jim Rohn

Learn about nutrition. Get the facts about fats, sugars, carbohydrates and sodium and read every food label and nutritional breakdown.

Know the impact on your body when you digest, for example, a 12 ounce soda that contains 39 grams of sugar.   Realize when you are ingesting over 3500mg. of sodium in one order of barbeque ribs so there's no shock in the morning when your eyes bug out and your fingers swell, not to mention what it does to your blood pressure!

Why shouldn't you use your power and kick victim-hood in the butt. No more lack of awareness; no more allowing mindless behavior and blaming it on your genes.

Take control and make conscious well-informed choices. If you really want something, have it fully aware of the consequences.   Live in partnership with yourself and take charge of making your own choices in awareness. Fat genes or not, it's still you making the choices. It's still you who can exercise control.

32. Think positively because everything flows from your thoughts.

If you're unhappy and dissatisfied, acknowledge it and initiate the one-piece rule. Think about your life right now and ask yourself what one improvement could make you feel better? How and where could you begin to make a change, a step in the right direction?

Know your mind and your emotions. Learn to ask self-reflective questions, discerning questions, probing questions that reveal more of yourself. Then help yourself with self knowledge to shift and change what you can control. The more you know about yourself, the more you can develop self-support and help.

The simple step of taking action is therapy but it has to be the right action, one that you have chosen from awareness of what you want, what you don't want, and why.

Reflect on your friends and decide if they are a bridge to your goals or a barrier. Negative friends will bring you down because that is how negative influences operate. Notice the energy profile of your friends, how they behave, how they speak, how they live and decide if they pull you upwards towards growth and empowerment, or hold you in mediocrity or worse.

33. **Read self-help books and listen to audios** that give you encouragement and momentum to change your life. Remember what you want and why you want it. Keep feeding your mind what it needs to hear.   Positive talks, reading and expressions will empower you and everyone needs to reinforce what works. Positive input cultivates success. Success takes work and it's your responsibility to live your best life possible.

34. Develop a warrior mindset.

You will not give up your habits without a battle. You know your place and what to expect even if you don't like what you get. You feel safe and comfortable with the status quo. Changing it will not come easily or quickly but it will come with perseverance.

Every fiber of your being will resist efforts to change one iota of yourself. It's your two wolves.

Care to read about your two wolves?

"A Tale of Two Wolves"   --unknown author

"An old Cherokee was teaching his grandchildren about life.

He told them about a battle that was raging inside him.

He said to them,

A battle is raging inside me. It is a terrible fight between two wolves.

One wolf represents fear, anger, envy, regret, greed, arrogance, self-pity, guilt,,

jealousy, inferiority, lies, false pride, and ego.

The other stands for joy, peace, love, happiness, harmony, humility,

kindness, friendship, empathy, generosity, truth, compassion, forgiveness and

faith."

The old man fixed his eyes upon the children with a firm stare.

"The same fight is going on inside you, and inside every other

person too."

The children thought about it for a minute and then one child

asked his grandfather, "which wolf will win?"

The old Cherokee replied, ".the one you feed."

Which wolf will you feed?

You have a decision to make right now. You can either use this information and take action, small consistent action, or not.

If you understand the division within your own self, one wanting changes desperately, the other fighting changes desperately to keep you the same, your choice becomes which wolf.

The thoughts you choose feed only one wolf. Which wolf will you feed? It is your decision.

35. Small hinges swing big doors. Small changes bring big rewards.

____Suggested small changes to start:

- Eliminate fruit drinks and juices. (Loaded with sugar!)

- Give up second helpings.

- Start walking every day.

- Take the stairs everywhere possible.

- Skip snacks and nibbling in between meals.

- If you're hungry between meals, eat protein, or fruit, say no to fried foods, dessert snacks and energy bars. (no matter the claim of good health. They are high impact high calorie/carbohydrates/sugar foods.

- Eat fresh vegetables, steamed, micro-waved, boiled, plain no butter, no cream sauces. Get back to the basics of simple foods.

- Try lemon. Try pepper and salt, fresh lemon.

- No sampling free food or drinks. (Nothing is free. It costs you.)

- Forget store bought muffins or donuts. Check their nutritional footprint! It is big. One slice of lemon cake at Starbucks, almost 500 calories. Wow! What else could you eat for 500 calories that would be more substantial and fulfilling? Lots.

- Give up junk food. Choose healthier baked snacks. Read labels.

- Give up fried foods. Try baked, steamed, sautéed, grilled.

- If you can't avoid fried, remove the fried batter from your meal. With chicken, skin it and eat the protein by itself. If it's fish, ditto the batter and eat only the fish. Try it.

- Drain anything fried. Blot with napkins. Leave some. Skin it.

- Check food labels for sugar or sucrose content and avoid foods that have high gram counts per serving.

- 4 grams of sugar or sucrose equals 16 calories or one teaspoon. (Every 4 grams of sugar = one teaspoon in the product.)

- Labels with fructose, corn sweeteners, honey, maple syrup, molasses, sorbitol, amazake, turbinado, dextrose, carob powder, high fructose corn syrup, beet sugar, brown and cane sugars, all relate to the sweet stuff so be aware. (4gr. to 1 ratio)

- Eliminate soda and soft drinks. They're loaded with sugar and deplete your body of calcium. Diet drinks deplete calcium too. Big time issues for women.

- Be aware of carbohydrate overload. Set maximum intake for yourself.

- Fresh fruit will help relieve sugar cravings.

- Drink natural juices like carrot.

- Drink water with a squeeze of fresh lemon. The lemon is a natural ph balancer in your body. Try carbonated water or seltzer and club soda.

- Cut down on highly salted foods, read content labels on all canned goods, baked goods, restaurant foods which now provide nutritional information upon request. Get it. Know the consequences of your choices.

- Eliminate frozen baked goods, pies, frosted cakes,high in fat, sugar & carbohydrates.

- Give up mochas, frappuchinos, macchiatos and other high calorie high sugar fruit and yogurt drinks. Carrot juice works.

- Fresh squeezed orange juice too.

- Control gravies on meats and potatoes by getting it served on the side. Dizzle it on yourself. Ditto butter on your bread; get it on the side. How about syrup on pancakes? You do it.

- Get dressings, gravies, sauces and syrups brought on the side. Order your food plain with every thing served on the side. Then you can control the amount you eat.

  Otherwise, you're giving up your power to an outside source that cares nothing about your weight, health, looks or future. Don't give away your power. You take control and do everything yourself. You can have everything you want, but not drowning in gobs of high calorie high fat sauces that come naturally in restaurant servings. Exercise your judgment.

- Avoid all you can eat restaurants. They are an invitation to gluttony.

36. Upgrade your awareness.

Ask yourself questions every day.

"How can I choose to have a good day today?"

Ask it when you wake each day and throughout the day as challenges or stress arises.

Remember, it's a choice and your choices create your life.

Pause to choose better, smarter, in power, one decision at a time. It's the power of one.

Remember to ask:

"Is this moving me closer to the life I want or further away?"

"Am I happy"

"Is eating this helping me or hurting me?"

37. **Pause for reflections**. Any time, anywhere, pause and ask yourself what you are doing? Determine, is this what you REALLY want? Are you willing to make a different choice? Are you willing to try?

38. Pause every day often and acknowledge the person you are, just as you are and intend self-friendship, compassion, help, because anything less, keeps you in the space of punishment and judgment.

You don't have to like your behavior and you can agree to change it, but you do have to like who you are at your core. Behavior can be changed.

If you don't like any part of it, you have the power to change some or all of it with your choices. Make your plans, take action. Remember the power of one. Reflect and recall that you are that power. You alone.

39. **Be proactive**. Say mantras repeatedly throughout the day. Feed yourself positive energy. Tell yourself what you need to hear. Reinforce your desire and motivation to change your life. Thoughts occupy your mind incessantly so take charge of them. Grow them positively. Notice them. Change them. Direct them.

- "Today is a brand new day with brand new opportunities."

- "Today I will choose and make decisions that serve me."

- "Today I will eat better and healthier foods."

- "Today I will be more active to burn calories."

- "Today I create a positive environment and stay aware of my choices. All my choices have consequences and better choices promote my happiness."

Upgrading your awareness with self-attention brings increased self-accountability. Otherwise, mindless eating will persist. After all, if you miss the details of eating, then it's not your fault, is it when the bag is empty?

40. <u>WIZARD'S Wisdom</u>

The "go on, go off" diet message holds an unrealistic promise of change. And it sets women up to fail in the day-to-day management of their lives when they switch "off" their diet, untutored, unskilled and weak in managing old habits that return and get them and keep them fat!

Women need a strategic base rooted in a mindset that approaches weight management as an integral part of their behavior every day, and not only when it's an emergency 911 action.

Your lifestyle yesterday, today, tomorrow affects who you are, how you feel and how you look. Growing overweight is the cumulative affect of all your actions, one calorie at a time, one decision at a time, one ounce at a time, one pound at a time. It's as simple as that! All your choices matter every day, every choice.

Open your mind to diet as your <u>style of living, your lifestyle, what you do every day, every meal, every snack, every nibble</u>. It all matters, it all contributes to the big picture of your life adding extra calories and weight, or not; managing effectively or not.

Live that idea. Live your diet every day and practice smarter choices, practice self-awareness and practice any or all of Wizard's 50 ways to change your life with strategies to win. Do one, some or all and get involved with owning all your time; get active with unveiling the illusion of "on/off" diets so you can live with yourself every day in cooperation rather than in battle.

Learn, Practice, Develop Discernment Skills

See yourself, pay attention to yourself and notice what you think and how you feel. If you are having a bad day, can you agree to reason with yourself and try to diffuse whatever has you down? Try to get over it quickly so it doesn't drive you to 911-food.   How can you make a situation less toxic so it doesn't send you binging? Ask yourself questions. How will eating make your life better? It won't. It changes nothing. Only you can change you, only you can help you. So try it.

41. **Practice trend watching.** Think about your day as you go through the day and notice the trend of your thoughts and Where it takes you. Do you complain, criticize, judge, regret, envy more than not? Be honest. Are your friends and associates negative, griping queens, or gossip prone? These are eating outlets, every one, and you need to see how pervasive negative thought patterns are to a balanced relationship with food.

The environment inside your minds affects your behavior, your attitude and your choices. You can influence your behavior by influencing your thoughts once you pay attention to them. If you want to feel positive and happier, cultivate your mind to attract it by upgrading your thoughts and what you think about. Focus on things, people, circumstances and ideas that make you feel good. Resist the complainer in yourself and in others, resist attention on what's missing, focus on positives and change your attitude.

42. Be your own best friend. Have a heart to heart talk with yourself as a friend, as you would guide and support a sister, a family member, a person about whom you care. Stay the course, even when you may be off your game and may be overeating, just pick yourself up and start again with better insights than before about what didn't work. Ask yourself:

> "How can I do better next time?"
>
> "How can I be more effective?"
>
> "What brought me down?"
>
> "What's a more positive approach for me?"
>
> "What did I learn and how can I use it to help myself?"

43. Use power words that enable your intentions, and help you stay the course. Feed yourself positive ideas:

> "I can do this"
>
> "I am capable"
>
> "I am powerful and can always make a better choice."
>
> "I am doing my best and my best is all there is."

44.   Develop Risk Management skills.

See the risk in shopping when you are hungry.

See it in <u>not</u> reading and <u>not</u> understanding food labels.

Realize "free" food snacks or "samples" NOT free. You pay.

Recognize:

- Boredom, disappointment, routine-rut and stress.

- Overwhelm and doing it all syndrome.

- Wasting time and non-productive diversions.

- Not delegating, not making demands, no expectations.

- No personal boundaries. No professional boundaries.

- No time for yourself.

- No outlets for yourself except eating.

- Not speaking up for yourself without guilt.

- Not defining what you want and why.

- Not accepting your own right to a life.

- Not writing your goals and habit reform plan.

- Not implementing daily routines to support you.

- Not practicing awareness.

- Not having any fun.

- Once you identify at risk behavior, you can change it and help protect yourself from self-entrapment.

45. Read motivational books, articles, self-help programs, and videos. Search Google for Will Smith, the actor, and be inspired. Search Google for Randy Pausch and listen to his last lecture and open your heart to what matters.

Use mental hugs and kisses by supporting yourself every way possible. Talk to yourself, help yourself, love yourself.

46. Set and reset and adjust small achievable goals. Live the power of one and wake up every day with the intention of making one improvement in your behavior. Just one. One every day added to the next and the next and your entire life is upgraded by the power of one. You are that power.

47. Review your life every day, not as a judge or critic or complainer but as an observer. What did you observe and what did you learn from it? Do you like the behavior? Do you not like the behavior and how do you envision changing it? What steps would help you get a better more acceptable result?

48.   Knowledge is power but without action, it's dormant. Live your power. Take action. Use your mind to think about right action and how you can better manage your life and your eating. Take small steps to eat smarter and implement a lifestyle of self-management that works for you. Live your knowledge, grow your knowledge.

49.   "Pity the man who has a favorite restaurant but not a favorite author. He's picked out a favorite place to feed his body but he doesn't have a favorite place to feed his mind."
Words of ---   Jim Rohn

50. Change Your Strategy and Change Your Results.

Listen to your heart, get in touch with you inner self to reset your intentions to know and serve the person you truly are, and empower your life with small proactive actions.

What would you like to create for yourself?

One step taken is one step closer.   You are the only person who can take the actions necessary to change what it is you want to change.

Congratulations to you! And my best wishes to you always.

Contact information: rosemaryhershey@gmail.com